HERBS FOR DETOXIFICATION

Pathway to Robust Health

KAREN BRADSTREET

WOODLAND PUBLISHING
Pleasant Grove, UT

© 1997
Woodland Publishing, Inc.
P.O. Box 160
Pleasant Grove, UT
84062

The information in this book is for educational purposes only and is not recommended as a means of diagnosing or treating an illness. All matters concerning physical and mental health should be supervised by a health practitioner knowledgeable in treating that particular condition. Neither the publisher nor author directly or indirectly dispense medical advice, nor do they prescribe any remedies or assume any responsibility for those who choose to treat themselves.

TABLE OF CONTENTS

THE MAGIC OF DETOXIFICATION	5
THE NEED FOR DETOXIFICATION	6
THE DANGER OF TOXIC OVERLOAD	7
ORIGINS OF DETOXIFICATION	8
THE ROLE OF HERBS AND SUPPLEMENTS	9
WHEN TO DETOXIFY	10
HOW TO GO ON A DETOXIFICATION PROGRAM	11
WHAT TO EXPECT ON A DETOXIFICATION PROGRAM	12
ORGANS OF DETOXIFICATION AND ELIMINATION	14
THE LIVER AND KIDNEYS	14
THE COLON	19
THE BLOOD AND LYMPHATIC SYSTEM	24
DETOXIFYING HERBS REFERENCE GUIDE	28
REFERENCES	31

THE MAGIC OF DETOXIFICATION

Imagine finding a body potion that could wash away the damaging effects of junk foods, environmental pollutants, and other things that rob us of vitality. Gone from cells, organs and fat pockets would be the residues of glazed donuts, potato chips, beefsteaks and soft drinks. Every cell in the body would be pulsating with renewed life.

Unfortunately, no such potion exists. But, there is something that can work like magic in building health, something that numerous cultures have used throughout history for cleansing and physical renewal. That something is a simple and natural process called detoxification.

Detoxification—sometimes called blood purification or body cleansing—is the practice of altering dietary habits to give the body's eliminative channels a chance to get rid of toxins in cells, organs, tissues, the bloodstream and the lymphatic system.

In practice, detoxification is accomplished by abstaining from food for a few hours or days (fasting), drinking only juices, taking special herbs, or any combination of a number of methods to give the body a chance to divert its energies from digesting food to detoxifying and renewing itself.

THE NEED FOR DETOXIFICATION

Good health is the sum total of many different parts. Consider how your current state of health is a reflection of the following things:

1) What you take into your body—the quality of your food and drink, and the air you breathe. The body is designed to handle some toxins, but can become overloaded when bombarded with processed foods, air pollutants, and beverages loaded with chemical additives and stimulants.

2) Elimination—the effectiveness of organs designed to eliminate waste matter, including the colon, kidneys, liver and lymphatic system. If the channels of elimination aren't flowing freely, toxic buildup is inevitable and one's health will suffer.

3) Circulation—the frequency of exercise and movement. Exercise helps the body eliminate toxic buildup through perspiration and stimulation of the eliminative organs.

4) Emotional and spiritual health—whether you suffer from chronic negative emotions such as worry, anger, or have a positive outlook and spiritual well-being. Negative emotions can be toxic to physical health. Cleansing the emotions is as vital to health as cleansing the body.

5) Inheritance—the genetic code you received from your parents. You may be stuck with your genes, but with attention to items 1-4 above, it's possible to overcome some inherited weaknesses.

The human body is in a constant state of renewal, a process of old cells dying and new ones taking their place. The entire body rebuilds in less than two years, and 98 percent rebuilds in less than a year. Blood takes about four months to regenerate, the liver six weeks, the skin one month, and the stomach lining only five days.

You can literally transform your health by working with your body's natural regeneration process. But before the body can rebuild healthy tissues and organs, it must first be cleansed of toxic materials. If it is not, the natural renewal process will be overwhelmed. Even when you eat the best of foods, if your body is burdened with toxins and mucus you'll fail to get optimal results. It is important to begin almost any health program with a good detoxification program, and undertake a periodic detoxification program throughout your lifetime.

The Danger of Toxic Overload

The dangerous effect of toxic buildup in the body is eloquently stated by Dr. Ross Trattler in *Better Health Through Natural Healing*.

> Accumulation of toxic material within the body due to improper diet, poor circulation, poor elimination, and lack of demanding exercise is a major factor in almost all disease. While it is acknowledged that other causes do exist, most factors that predispose to disease result in an accumulation of poisonous substances in the body which, when the channels of elimination cannot adequately remove them, will invariably initiate a disease process. These accumulations ultimately lead to changes within the cell and eventually within the whole body.

Many health problems can be improved through detoxification, from simple illnesses such as allergies, to more serious diseases like cancer. Regular detoxification is also an effective way to prevent many diseases from occurring. Edward Shook, one of the 21st century's most renowned natural healers, explains well the importance of detoxification in his book *Advanced Treatise in Herbology* (p. 33).

> The herbalist and natural healer . . . recognizes that disease, excluding trauma, is the result of the violation, intentional or otherwise, of the laws of nature; that germs cannot exist in harmful numbers for any length of time in or on tissue whose

life and vitality is so high that the only way the disease can be overcome is to aid nature in the healing process by the elimination of the poisons and toxins through the body's natural channels and allowing the vitality to return to its normal strength. In other words, disease is not cured by adding poisons to the body, but by eliminating them and observing the laws of nature, aiding and assisting her in every possible way.

The body absorbs toxins through the digestive system, lungs and skin. Sources of toxicity include:

- Waste products in the blood from illness or disease
- Smog, industrial pollutants, chemical fumes, car exhaust
- Food preservatives, dyes
- Household cleansers
- Poor elimination of food
- Normal metabolic processes

ORIGINS OF DETOXIFICATION

The practice of periodic detoxification goes far back in recorded history. Hippocrates, considered the father of modern medicine, made references to it. Health traditions as diverse as those of the of the Chinese, Asiatic Indians, and Europeans practiced various cleansing methods. Virtually all forms of traditional medicine—from Ayurveda to Chinese to Native American—still practice some form of detoxification. Fasting (abstaining from food and/or drink), a part of many religions around the world, is also a form of both physical and spiritual detoxification.

European immigrants brought cleansing practices to America with them. For instance, the Pennsylvania Germans (often nicknamed the Pennsylvania Dutch) ate wild greens like dandelion, lettuce, plantain and other herbs in the spring to cleanse their bodies after a long winter of heavy foods. Shaker herbal recipes include concoctions they call the "pukes" to purify the blood during the spring.

Native American tribes also practiced cleansing. Tribes in the Southwest used a black tea made from yaupon holly (*Ilex vomitoria*) that was considered sacred. Depending on the strength and dose, the tea could produce vomiting, sweating and profuse bowel evacuation. The tea was used in a variety of rituals, including spring cleaning.

The practice of detoxification is no less important to people in various lands today. For instance, in France today many use a tea called Tisane Provençal, a special blend of herbs designed to cleanse the liver, kidneys, bowels, and the body in general. It is available at any French drugstore.

Nature herself seems to suggest the importance of detoxification. Many of the plants that burst forth in early spring are cleansing in nature. Dandelion greens, for example, are high in minerals and other substances that cleanse the urinary system. Cherries, an early spring fruit, have a definite cleansing effect on the bowels and also eliminate uric acid buildup (linked to heavy meat consumption and considered a primary cause of gout and joint problems).

Those who lived before the development of modern food processing and refrigeration, people who lived in harmony with the earth's natural cycles, noticed the action these springtime foods had on their bodies. The wonderful feeling of cleansing after a winter of eating heavy foods was incentive enough for the practice of cleansing to take hold.

THE ROLE OF HERBS AND SUPPLEMENTS

Almost like a magic potion, herbs and other supplements can cleanse the body of toxic matter. Herbs contain a wide variety of natural compounds, often referred to as phytonutrients, that have many different cleansing actions. Some, such as cascara sagrada, encourage bowel elimination and help cleanse waste matter that may have accumulated over weeks, months or even years. Others, like the common herb yarrow, encourage sweating to eliminate toxins. Herbs such as wormwood and pumpkin seed cleanse the body of health-robbing parasites. Several herbs are diuretics—they encourage urination and have a cleansing effect on the urinary system. Various other herbs stimulate the liver to release toxins, thereby cleansing and restoring health to this vital protective organ. Many herbs have a general cleansing effect, while others target specific organs.

Unlike drugs, herbs work with normal body processes. Rather than mask symptoms, they help provide the raw materials—vitamins, minerals, enzymes, and unique chemical compounds—with which the body can cleanse and heal itself. The effectiveness and general safety of herbs is one reason people are turning to herbal medicine in record numbers. Many other natural supplements are available that work well with herbs in detoxifying the body. You'll find recommendations in this booklet to help you develop your own cleansing program.

When to Detoxify

The body sends obvious signals when it is suffering from toxic overload, but you need not wait until symptoms appear to go on a detoxification program. In fact, the ideal time to make detoxification a regular practice is before symptoms occur. However, human nature being what it is, most people wait until they have health problems before examining their health habits. The good news is that it's never too late—and better late than never! Signs of toxicity include:

- Fatigue
- Constipation
- Offensive breath
- Low immunity
- Hormone imbalances
- Nausea
- Gas
- Dizziness
- Poor circulation
- Depression, mood swings
- PMS
- Mucus buildup
- Skin problems (acne, eczema, dryness, itchiness)

If warning signs are ignored, eventually full-blown disease is almost inevitable. Ideal times to detoxify are:

- When you suffer from any of the aforementioned symptoms
- In the spring
- Before going on a weight-loss program
- After a period of poor eating, such as the holidays or a vacation
- When you are in generally good health, not weakened by a serious disease
- Anytime you feel your body could use a break from poor eating habits

How to Go on a Detoxification Program

A detoxification program can last as long as you feel necessary—anywhere from two or three days to a couple of weeks or longer, depending on your health goal. If you simply feel sluggish and would like to give your body a jump-start, a shorter cleanse will usually accomplish your goals. If you're suffering from a serious illness or disease, you may need to detoxify for an extended period of time, or detoxify in cycles, with rest periods in between. A feeling of renewal and well-being is the sign you've accomplished your goal.

General Guidelines

- A day or two before you officially begin your detoxification program, make sure you eat a light diet of wholesome foods such as raw fruits, vegetables, and whole grains to begin gentle cleansing. You may also drink only juices for a day or two, although this is not recommended during the winter months in cold climates because it hampers the body's production of energy and heat.
- Eliminate all toxic substances from your diet including coffee, tea, chocolate, soda, tobacco, artificial colorings and flavorings, white

sugar, white flour, red meat, and any and all kinds of other junk foods. Stick to fresh fruits and vegetables, whole grains, raw nuts, and other natural foods. The higher the quality of food you eat, the better your body will be able to detoxify and rebuild.
- Frequently use a sauna or jacuzzi. They can help the body sweat out poisons, many of which accumulate in body fat.
- Use herbs. Because individual responses to cleansing vary, this booklet cannot recommend specific herb amounts. For the herbs suggested, follow label directions or consult with the product supplier or distributor for guidance.

What to Expect on a Detoxification Program

Healing Crisis

Many people are surprised to find that when they begin a detoxification program, they initially feel worse than ever. This is because the body is releasing toxins that have accumulated in organs and tissues into the bloodstream for elimination. If this happens, be confident your body is functioning exactly the way nature designed. You may experience flu-like symptoms, including profuse mucus production, body chills or aches, headaches and diarrhea. This reaction is known as a healing crisis. If you experience the symptoms described, hang in there. When it is over, you'll feel better than ever. A healing crisis:

- Happens as the body is cleansed through fasting, semi-fasting, and building or cleansing herbs and foods.
- Happens only if the body has enough vitality to stand the shock.
- Happens when a person feels the best.
- Usually takes about three months of correct eating to bring about a healing crisis; may come sooner when fasting.

- Usually only lasts two or three days.
- Sometimes no crisis occurs because the body eliminates waste gradually.
- Normally, the body only cleanses to the point where it can tolerate poisonous waste. During a healing crisis, however, the body completely eliminates toxic buildup.

Some cleansing programs, such as those using mild herbs, are designed for slow cleansing, and may not cause symptoms. A gentler cleansing method is appropriate for those in weakened health, whose bodies cannot easily withstand the shock of a healing crisis. In such cases, it is better to first build up the body's strength with supplements and healthy foods. When strength returns, gentle cleansing can begin. If the body tolerates gentle cleansing well, one can begin a more concentrated cleansing program.

Disease Crisis

As mentioned earlier, people who suffer from severe toxic buildup or chronic disease may be too weak to experience a healing crisis. People in this category may experience what is referred to as a disease crisis. A disease crisis:

- Happens when the body is clogged with mucus.
- Happens when strength and vitality are at a low point.
- Saves life. If toxic buildup continues, the body's protective mechanisms could be overcome and disease would result.
- Lasts several weeks.

Remember, if you feel worse after beginning a detoxification program, don't give up. It is a sign your body is releasing toxins into the bloodstream for elimination. Stick with it. You WILL feel better when it's over!

ORGANS OF DETOXIFICATION AND ELIMINATION

No discussion of detoxification would be complete without mentioning the organs of elimination. Detoxification programs target organs whose role is to cleanse and protect the body from toxic substances—primarily the liver and kidneys, colon, and lymphatic and blood system. Detoxification can target each of these organs individually, or all of them together.

If you have a known weakness with a certain body organ, you should follow the general cleansing guidelines offered earlier in this booklet, and select herbs and supplements that target the particular organ you need to focus on. For instance, if you have symptoms of liver weakness, such as acne or a hormone imbalance, select herbs and supplements that cleanse and build the liver, including milk thistle and dandelion root.

If you would like to undertake a general detoxification program, look for combinations of herbs and vitamins designed for general cleansing (look in the herb reference section at the end of this booklet for suggestions). Many companies offer herbal combinations specifically designed for general detoxification.

THE LIVER AND KIDNEYS

Among its 500 plus functions, the liver plays a key role in converting toxic substances into nontoxic substances. These conversions are performed primarily by enzymes that break down toxins into less toxic substances, which are then excreted by the kidneys. Both the liver and the kidneys must be functioning properly to protect us from toxins.

Because the liver plays so many roles in protecting health, when it is overburdened with toxins, health problems may arise in any of the areas related to liver function—energy production, blood sugar regulation, and hormone production and regulation. A hormone imbalance, for instance, is usually a sign of a malfunctioning or overburdened liver.

A wide variety of toxins impair the ability of these enzymes to do their jobs. Such toxins include almost all prescription and nonprescription drugs (including birth control pills and Prozac), food additives (including many dyes and preservatives), and environmental toxins (paint fumes, car exhaust, etc.). Nutritional deficiencies can also impair the function of these enzymes. When the liver becomes overloaded with toxic substances that it cannot neutralize, disease is inevitable. In reference to this, naturopathic physician Dan Lukaczer says:

> Over the past ten years, extensive research has shown that sluggish, imbalanced or impaired detoxification systems can cause accumulation and deposition of metabolic toxins, impairing the energy production of cells and increasing free-radical production . . . The relative detoxification ability of an individual plays an important role in susceptibility or resistance to the toxicity or carcinogenicity of specific substances. Research has shown that detoxification rates may be predictive for certain cancers.

Dr. Lukaczer goes on to suggest a link between the liver's ability to detoxify and chronic fatigue syndrome, Parkinson's disease, Alzheimer's disease, lupus and rheumatoid arthritis. He cites cases of using nutritional support to boost the body's detoxifying process, with significant improvement. For example, vitamin C is especially important to liver function. In one study, guinea pigs deprived of vitamin C for only a few days showed reduced ability to break down chemicals.

Dietary Recommendations for Liver and Kidney Detoxification

Don'ts:

- Avoid the use of all drugs, including alcohol and caffeine; avoid food additives and pesticides; avoid breathing polluted air and toxic fumes.

Dos:

- Eat plenty of fresh broccoli, cabbage, Brussels sprouts and cauliflower. These cruciferous vegetables contain sulfur compounds called glucosinolates, which have been studied for their anticancer potential. Part of their effectiveness may be in activating detoxifying enzymes.
- Consume adequate protein. Studies have shown the body's detoxification processes are hampered by inadequate protein intake.
- Try to breathe clean air and drink purified water.
- An ideal way to begin your liver detoxification program is with a three-day juice fast—drink only vegetable and fruit juices for three days.
- Fresh lemon juice in water is cleansing for the liver—drink several glasses daily.

A wide variety of herbs and supplements detoxify and build the liver and kidneys. Many companies offer herbal combinations specially designed to cleanse and rebuild the liver—look for combinations containing the ingredients below.

Herbs for Liver/Kidney Detoxification

Milk Thistle

This herb is essential in any program designed to build liver health. Its benefits are documented by extensive research. Milk thistle increases the production of a substance called glutathione peroxidase in the liver, a powerful antioxidant that protects liver tissues and helps neutralize toxins. Milk thistle also regenerates damaged liver tissue.

DANDELION ROOT

Dandelion root contains bitter substances that stimulate the liver and kidneys to release toxins. It is high in vitamin A, a nutrient particularly important to liver function.

BARBERRY ROOT BARK

Barberry was traditionally prescribed by 19th century eclectic physicians as a cure for jaundice, a disease caused by too much bile in the blood. The root is high in iron, selenium and calcium.

TURMERIC

Turmeric holds an esteemed place in Ayurvedic medicine as an overall body cleanser. It contains an antioxidant called curcumin, shown in animal studies to protect liver tissue exposed to liver-damaging drugs.

BURDOCK ROOT

Burdock is a traditional herb for treating cancer. In studies done with animals, burdock has demonstrated a protective effect against toxic chemicals.

KELP

Kelp exerts a powerful protective effect against toxins. It contains a chemical called sodium alginate which protects the body from radiation exposure and heavy metal toxicity. Animals fed sodium alginate reduced their absorption of strontium-90 (a toxic heavy metal released in nuclear accidents) by as much as 83 percent. Other studies show that kelp protects the body from absorbing the toxic metals barium, cadmium, plutonium and cesium.

Parsley

As a diuretic, parsley encourages urination and has a gentle laxative effect. These actions are attributed to the chemicals apiol and myristicin. It is traditionally used to treat jaundice.

Rose Hips

Hips contain a significant amount of vitamin C which is essential to healthy liver function.

Other Supplements

Vitamins A, C, E, and B-Complex; Minerals; Zinc and Selenium

These are all powerful antioxidants that protect the liver from damage, neutralize toxic substances and provide necessary nutrients.

Free-form Amino Acids

Free-form amino acids build the liver and are easily utilized because they are already broken down.

Coenzyme Q-10

Co Q-10 supplies the liver with oxygen and has a protective effect.

Lecithin

Lecithin prevents fat buildup in the liver.

Freeze-dried Cruciferous vegetables

Freeze-dried vegetables contain raw materials that help the liver build enzymes used to detoxify harmful substances.

THE COLON

"Health begins in the colon" is a common saying among natural health advocates. This statement is based on the fact that the colon is the body's main channel of elimination. But the fact is that modern Western society is plagued with diet-related colon problems. More than 20 percent of Americans suffer from constipation. From irritable bowel to colitis to colon cancer, we endure problems unknown in countries where high-fiber diets are a way of life. It is no coincidence that laxatives are one of today's top-selling non-prescription drugs.

People in third world countries consume about two and a half times more fiber than those in Western countries. Standard transit time for food in the colon is eighteen hours in undeveloped nations, whereas in the United States, food transit time can take from three days to two weeks. Speaking of the dangers of slow elimination, Warren Levin, a holistic physician, says, "If the bowel content is small, it can take from 75 to 100 hours for the foods we eat to pass through. When this occurs, there is stagnation and putrefaction. Foods become toxic and we absorb toxins. This is one of the ways in which ill health is produced . . . ."

Processed grains such as white flour and white rice, fast food, and prepackaged foods inhibit the normal elimination process. These foods lack the fiber needed to move waste matter through the large intestine for elimination. They also contain dozens of unhealthy ingredients like preservatives, dyes, and unhealthy fats which contribute to constipation. Such foods create small, hard stools that have a long transit time in the colon and are difficult to eliminate.

If food is allowed to sit in the colon for long periods of time it becomes a breeding ground for toxins that poison the whole body. This phenomenon is called autointoxication, or self-poisoning. Many diseases begin in an unhealthy colon when toxins are allowed to stagnate and spread to other organs and tissues. For that reason, colon cleansing is always a good way to begin a detoxification program.

A healthy colon eliminates remnants of undigested food, secretions from the intestines such as mucus and salt, and bacteria and parasites that are broken down from blood and tissues. In recent years it has been verified that healthy elimination can even prevent diseases such as breast cancer, and that a fiber-rich diet—essential to healthy elimination—lowers cholesterol and thereby plays a role in preventing heart disease. Every function of the body is in some way influenced by the health of the colon. Obviously then, periodic colon detoxification not only eliminates accumulated fecal matter, but it also allows for optimal absorption of nutrients.

Dietary Recommendations for Colon Detoxification

DON'TS:
- Avoid caffeine, white rice, fast and prepackaged foods, red meat and products containing white flour and sugar. If you are lactose intolerant, avoid milk products.

DOS:
- Raw, fresh fruits and vegetables, whole grains, brown rice and legumes provide fiber needed for healthy elimination.
- Generally speaking, most people can benefit from a colon cleanse twice yearly. A colon detoxification program should include: 1) herbs that act as loosening agents for cleansing, 2) bulking agents to assist elimination, and 3) absorbing agents to pull out toxins. In addition, herbs that promote peristalsis (the intestinal action that causes food to be eliminated), herbs or supplements that build the colon's supply of healthy bacteria, and antigas agents round out a complete colon program. Refer to the end of this section for recommended herbs and supplements.
- If you feel miserable and/or have severe persistent diarrhea during an intestinal cleanse, you may be cleansing too fast and should try cutting back on some of your supplements or use milder herbs.

- To speed up the cleansing action, try fasting while doing an herbal cleanse. When you stop eating, your body quickly eliminates mucus, fats, and toxic buildup. Most people should not fast more than three to ten days (using liquids) without supervision.
- Exercise is essential to colon health. Exercise speeds up bowel action and encourages healthy elimination.

Be patient—most improvements don't happen immediately, although they can. One woman who had suffered from colitis for four years began using psyllium hulls to cleanse her colon and digestive enzymes to help with food digestion. She experienced complete healing in two weeks, with no recurrence even years later. Other cases may take patient cycles of cleansing and building, but the results can be dramatic. Increased vitality will definitely come.

Many companies offer combinations containing herbs and other supplements designed to both detoxify and nourish the colon. Look for combinations containing the ingredients that follow.

Herbs for Colon Detoxification

CASCARA SAGRADA BARK

One of the world's most popular medicinal herbs, cascara sagrada is a laxative of unparalleled value. It is found in dozens of over-the-counter laxatives and is essential in any colon-detoxification program. Cascara contains chemicals called anthraquinones that stimulate bowel elimination. The herb also works to restore bowel tone. Cascara is highly effective but milder than many other laxative herbs such as aloe, buckthorn, rhubarb and senna. It is less likely to cause intestinal discomfort and is ideal for widespread use.

BLACK WALNUT HULLS

High in iodine, black walnut hulls have value for any cleansing program because of their ability to kill intestinal parasites.

Psyllium Hulls

Psyllium offers two key benefits in a detoxification program. First, it provides bulk to help "scrub" the bowel clean, and second, it prevents the absorption of some toxic chemicals by carrying them out of the body before they cause damage. In one study, animals fed toxic food additives were protected from intestinal damage when givin psyllium hulls. Psyllium also lowers cholesterol by preventing its absorption in the colon. Psyllium can provide significant relief from constipation, hemorrhoids, irritable bowel syndrome, and other problems related to poor elimination.

Ginger Root

Ginger is as an antispasmodic that soothes the intestinal tract. It also prevents nausea, relieves indigestion and cramping in the intestine, and contains enzyme-type substances that help digest proteins.

Rhubarb Root

Rhubarb has been popular for centuries in China as a treatment for dysentery. Large amounts of rhubarb have a powerful laxative effect, a quality useful for any detoxification program. Its laxative action is due to chemicals called anthraquinones, similar to those in cascara sagrada, buckthorn and senna. Because of its strong action, rhubarb should not be used by those with ulcers or colitis. Do not use rhubarb for more than two weeks, as the body may develop a dependency on it.

Senna Leaves

Senna is one of the most powerful laxative herbs and should only be used in cases of severe constipation. Like other laxative herbs, it contains colon-stimulating chemicals called anthraquinones. It may cause intestinal cramping if too much is taken; however, small amounts of senna added to laxative herbal combinations should be no cause for concern.

Artemisia (Wormwood)

Many people today harbor intestinal parasites which secrete toxins and rob the body of vitality. Cleansing the body of parasites is an important part of any cleansing program. Artemisia is one of nature's best parasite eliminators. It also stimulates the liver and gallbladder.

Elecampane

Elecampane helps the body expel parasites, which are a root cause of many health problems including fatigue, flatulence, bloating, and other digestive problems. It contains a chemical called alantolactone that kills parasites, including pinworms and giardia. Elecampane can be taken alone or in combination with other herbs.

Garlic

Garlic is one of nature's most valuable gifts to humankind. As part of a cleansing program, garlic has powerful antibiotic properties. Along with other qualities too numerous to list here, garlic helps destroy the bacteria that cause tuberculosis, food poisoning, bladder infection, influenza, meningitis, athlete's foot, and yeast infections. It should be a component of any cleansing program.

Pumpkin Seeds

Pumpkin seeds are an effective cleanser of worms in both adults and children.

Goldenseal Root

Goldenseal contains two noteworthy chemicals, berberine and hydrastine, which kill many types of bacteria, fungi, and protozoa, including those that cause diarrhea, dysentery, giardia, and cholera. It also stimulates white blood cells, thereby boosting immunity.

Other Supplements

BENTONITE CLAY: Bentonine clay is highly absorptive and removes toxins from colon. It should only be used occasionally as it may deplete certain nutrients if overused.
LACTOBACILLUS ACIDOPHILUS: Acidophilus consists of healthy bacteria essential for colon health. Acidophilus bacteria manufacture B vitamins, keep unfriendly bacteria in check, and perform a host of other health-promoting activities. Unfortunately, acidphiolus is destroyed by antibiotics.
CHLOROPHYLL: Chlorophyll cleanses and detoxifies the body.
CHARCOAL: Charcoal is a powerful absorber of poisons, neutralizes toxins and absorbs excess gas in the colon.
CAPRYLIC ACID: This acid kills yeast which can inhabit the colon.
PEPSIN: Pepsin absorbs toxins and feeds the bowel.
APPLE PECTIN: Apple pectin absorbs toxins and soothes the bowel.

BLOOD AND LYMPHATIC SYSTEM

Although the concept of purifying the blood is ancient, it is as valid today as it was in times past. The bloodstream, working in partnership with the liver and kidneys, plays a vital role in cleansing our system of toxins and disease-causing agents.

Blood supplies life to all cells of the body. Without a pure blood supply, normal renewal cannot take place. Toxins carried by the blood to cells are often responsible for cellular deformation that eventually leads to diseased tissues and organs. Blood purifying herbs do not literally purify the blood. They work by stimulating the liver, kidneys, colon and/or lymphatic system, all of which are responsible for filtering toxins from the body for removal.

Dietary Recommendations for the Blood and Lymphatic System

Don'ts:

- Avoid products made with white flour and sugar, heated fats and oils (for at least a month), and all junk foods.

Dos:

- Drink plenty of purified water, fresh lemon juice, beet juice, carrot juice, dandelion tea. Drink at least eight glasses of water a day. Eat raw vegetables for several weeks, and drink green drinks often. Green drinks are made by blending vegetable greens (carrot tops, parsley, etc.) with pineapple juice in a blender.

Herbs for the Blood and Lymphatic System

Dandelion Root

Dandelion absorbs toxins, stimulates the liver and kidneys, and provides minerals to build health.

Yellow Dock

Considered a general blood purifier, yellow dock makes an excellent general tonic and cleanser. It is especially noted for use in treating skin problems, which are almost always a sign the body is trying to eliminate toxins through the skin.

Sarsaparilla Root

In 19th century America, syphilis was a widespread concern and sarsaparilla was a common treatment. This is one reason it has earned a reputation as a blood purifier. Sarsaparilla contains chemicals called saponins which act as diuretics.

Burdock Root

Cancer is often linked to toxins that disrupt normal cellular processes. Animal studies show that burdock prevents poisoning against toxic chemicals, and it is valued as a cancer treatment.

Echinacea Root

Echinacea is a powerful immune stimulant that kills a wide range of disease-causing viruses, protozoa, fungi and bacteria. It makes an excellent daily tonic.

Red Clover

Research has confirmed that red clover contains antitumor compounds, including daidzein and genistein. It also contains the antioxidant vitamin E. Red clover is considered a cancer treatment by as many as 33 different cultures worldwide.

Kelp

An essential part of any detoxification program, kelp has the remarkable ability to both detoxify the body and build health. It contains compounds that prevent the absorption of toxic metals and is a rich source of minerals.

Capsicum (Cayenne Pepper)

Capsicum stimulates blood circulation and is often added to herbal combinations as a catalyst.

Oregon Grape Root

Oregon grape contains the alkaloids hydrastine and berberine, also found in goldenseal. These phytonutrients have a cleansing and antibiotic effect.

Wheatgrass Juice

Wheat is considered the staff of life, but most wheat products consumed today have been highly refined and lost many of their valuable nutrients. Wheatgrass juice is exceptionally high in nutrients, is easily digested, and is invaluable in any detoxification/blood purification program.

PAU D'ARCO BARK

Pau d'arco is considered a blood purifier par excellence in South America and is often used as a cancer treatment. Its popularity has steadily increased in North America in recent years.

GOLDENSEAL ROOT

Goldenseal contains berberine and hydrastine, phytonutrients that have a powerful cleansing and antibiotic effect.

BUTCHER'S BROOM

Butcher's broom is recognized by herbalists as a cleanser for the circulatory system—it cleans arteries and is often used to treat varicose veins.

GARLIC

Cleansing for the entire body, garlic is of exceptional value for circulatory health. Studies published in the British journal *Lancet* document that garlic lowers cholesterol. It also prevents clotting that leads to heart attacks and reduces blood pressure. Garlic is a must-have in any cleansing program.

Other Supplements

OMEGA-3 OILS

Omega-3 oils feed and nourish the circulatory system. They may reverse the damage done by poor eating habits if taken along with a healthy diet of fresh fruits, vegetables and whole grains. They protect against plaque deposits which cause strokes, heart attacks and other heart ailments.

Coenzyme Q-10

This enzyme is part of the mitochondria of cells and is essential for energy production. It is beneficial for the entire circulatory system.

Vitamin C and Bioflavonoids

This family of nutrients are powerful detoxifiers, and are often recommended for those who use alcohol or drugs.

Chlorophyll

Chlorophyll is traditionally revered as a blood cleanser, but is also a great general detoxifier.

Detoxifying Herbs: A Reference Guide

There are many herbs with detetoxifying abilities. This guide will help you determine which herbs to use for your specific detoxification program.

General Cleansing Herbs

General cleansing herbs are good to use for when your vitality is low, or when you're in generally good health but feel a need to give your body a break from poor eating habits or a toxic environment. They should also be used when you're unsure of a particular organ to target or for preventive health care in a periodic detoxification program.

Garlic	Red clover
Burdock	Yellow dock
Nettle	Plantain
Sarsaparilla	Dandelion

Blood Purifiers (Alteratives)

Because the blood supplies life to all cells, tissues and organs, cleansing the blood improves the health of the whole body. Alterative herbs (such as those listed below) are most commonly used to treat toxic conditions such as acne and cancer that are created by blood impurities. They improve the blood, speed up elimination, improve digestion, and may increase appetite. Alteratives also increase the body's ability to eliminate toxins through the liver by enhancing bile flow. Some help eliminate toxins through the kidneys.

Burdock	Cat's claw (Uña de gato)
Dandelion	Oregon grape root
Pau d'Arco	Plantain
Red clover	Sarsaparilla
Yellow dock	Anthelmintics

The following alteratives help detoxify the body by killing parasites.

Aloe	Elecampane
Garlic	Pumpkin seed
Wormwood	

Cathartics

Cathartic herbs cause profuse bowel elimination and often stimulate bile secretion. They also help expel worms after an anthelmintic has been used. Rhubarb and senna are the two most common.

Diaphoretics

Diaphoretic herbs help detoxify the body by increasing perspiration, thus helping rid the body of toxins through the sweat glands. Their effects can be increased when taken as hot tea.

Blue vervain
Catnip
Ginger root
Spearmint

Boneset
Chamomile
Peppermint
Yarrow

Diuretics

Diuretic herbs increase the elimination of urine.

Bearberry
Burdock
Juniper
Yarrow

Buchu
Hydrangea
Parsley

Emmenagogues

Herbs which act as emmenagogues detoxify the female reproductive organs and may stimulate menstruation in some women.

Black cohosh
Cramp bark

Blue cohosh
False unicorn root

Laxatives

Laxative herbs help detoxification by encouraging bowel elimination. They are milder than purgatives and well-tolerated by most people.

Cascara sagrada
Psyllium hulls

Licorice root

Stimulants

Stimulant herbs increase circulation which, of course, is of overall benefit in cleansing.

Capsicum (cayenne)
Horseradish

Ginger root

REFERENCES

Balch, James E. and Phyills A. *Prescription for Nutritional Healing.* Garden City Park, NY: Avery Publishing Group, 1990.

Barney, Paul M.D. *Clinical Applications of Herbal Medicine.* Pleasant Grove, UT: Woodland Publishing, Inc., 1996.

Castleman, Michael. *The Healing Herbs.* Emmaus, PA: Rodale Press, 1991.

Griffith, H. Winter, M.D. *Complete Guide to Vitamins, Minerals and Supplements.* Tucson, AZ: Fisher Books, 1988.

Lust, John. *The Herb Book.* NY: Bantam Books, 1974.

Shook, Edward. *Advanced Treatise in Herbology.* Beaumont, CA: Trinity Center Press, 1978.

Tenney, Louise. *Health Handbook.* Pleasant Grove, UT: Woodland Publishing, Inc., 1987.